CW00734204

Lymphoe

Advice on self-m.......... and treatment

Peter Mortimer
MD, FRCP

Professor of Dermatological Medicine
to the University of London at St George's
and the Royal Marsden Hospitals

Jacquelyne Todd
PhD, MCSP, Graddipphys

Physiotherapist Consultant in Lymphoedema
Leeds Teaching Hospitals NHS Trust

THIRD EDITION

BEACONSFIELD PUBLISHERS LTD
Beaconsfield, Bucks, UK

First published 1988
Third edition 2007
Reprinted 2009, 2011

This book is copyright. All rights are reserved. Apart from any fair dealing for the purpose of private study, research, criticism or review, as permitted under the Copyright, Designs and Patents Act 1988, no part of this publication may be reproduced, stored or transmitted, in any form or by any means, without the prior permission in writing of the publishers. Enquiries should be addressed to Beaconsfield Publishers Ltd at 20 Chiltern Hills Road, Beaconsfield, Bucks HP9 1PL, UK.

books@beaconsfield-publishers.co.uk
www.beaconsfield-publishers.co.uk

© Peter Mortimer and Jacquelyne Todd 2007

The authors hereby assert their individual right as set out in sections 77 and 78 of the Copyright, Designs and Patents Act 1988 to be identified as the authors of this work wherever it is published commercially and whenever any adaptation of this work is published or produced.

British Library Cataloguing in Publication Data
    Mortimer, Peter, M.D.
    Lymphoedema : advice on self-management and treatment. –
    3rd ed.
      1.Lymphedema – Treatment – Popular works
      2.Self medication
      I. Title II.Todd, Jacquelyne III.Valentine, Jenny
      IV.Regnard, Claud F. B.
      616.4'2'06

    ISBN–10: 0–906584–59–0
    ISBN–13: 978–0–906584–59–0

Illustrations by Jenny Valentine
Phototypeset by Gem Graphics, Trenance, Mawgan Porth, Cornwall in 10¾ on 12½ Times.
Printed in Great Britain at Halstan & Co. Ltd, Amersham, Bucks.

Acknowledgements

The Lymphoedema Support Network (LSN) is a national charity committed to providing information for people with lymphoedema, their carers and their families. We would like to acknowledge the LSN's invaluable work in this field, and to thank them for helping to make this book a reality.

We would also like to record our thanks to Anita Wallace and her colleagues at the LSN, to Dr Vaughan Keeley and Anne Williams, and to Dr Caroline Badger, one of the co-authors of the previous version of this booklet, all of whom made the time to read various drafts of the manuscript, and whose thoughtful advice we were able to take into account when preparing the final version.

The royalties from the sale of this booklet are paid to three charities – Leeds Lymph Link, Breast Cancer Research Action Group, and Lymphoedema Support Network.

P.M., J.T.

CONTENTS

Contents

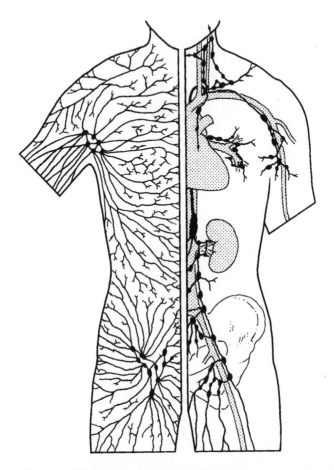

Figure 1: There are two parts to the lymph system. On the surface (shown on the left side) there are the lymph vessels and nodes beneath the skin. On the right side there are the deep vessels and nodes within the body.

INTRODUCTION

Lymphoedema is a swelling that arises because the lymph system is unable to work properly. It is a problem that can start at any time of life but is more common in older people. It can happen following treatment for cancer, although there can be other causes for the swelling. For many patients lymphoedema can be managed without too much difficulty, but in some cases the swelling needs more intensive treatment. A number of physical therapies used together on a regular basis are the most effective way to treat the condition. The use of drug therapy has had limited success, and surgery is not often a suitable treatment.

As it does not usually cause serious illness or pain and is rarely life-threatening, lymphoedema has often been regarded as a minor problem by doctors and health care managers. This has resulted in a shortage of treatment centres and skilled practitioners, and frustrating delays for people with the condition.

Despite recent advances there is still no treatment that will cure the problem and make it go away for good. But you can learn how to carry out some of the treatments that will help you to control your lymphoedema. This book describes why the problem develops and what can cause it to start. It then provides information about what the treatment involves and how you can help yourself.

THE LYMPH SYSTEM AND LYMPHOEDEMA

What is the lymph system?

The lymph system forms a network of drainage pathways around the body (Figure 1). It is an important way for extra fluid and waste products to be cleared away from cells and body tissues. The waste material passes back into the bloodstream and is eliminated from the body in the usual way. (The word 'tissues' as used in this booklet refers to a collection of similar cells in the body that work together to carry out the same function.)

The blood supplies every part of the body with water and proteins through tiny tubes (*blood vessels*) called *capillaries*. Fluid constantly passes through to the body tissues from blood capillaries. It is the *lymph vessels* that drain away this fluid (*lymph*) as well as the waste products produced by the body tissues. The lymph system forms an

1

overflow and waste disposal system for the body and is an important way for the tissues to stay healthy.

The smallest lymph vessels are called *initial lymphatics*. These tiny vessels work rather like a sponge to absorb fluid from the tissues. The lymph flows on through bigger vessels until it reaches special glands called *lymph nodes*. Parts of the body where groups of lymph nodes can be found are:

- neck
- armpits
- groin

The lymph nodes are an important part of the system, as it is here that water is absorbed back into the blood stream. They can filter out and break down any unwanted body products. More concentrated lymph flows on into large veins in the neck. The extra fluid that is not needed by the body is removed as urine and the blood recycles useful proteins.

The lymphatic system is an important part of the *immune system*, which is the body's main defence against infection. The lymph nodes contain *lymphocytes*, which are white cells found in both the blood and lymph system. These cells circulate through the body tissues and increase in number in the case of infection. This explains why lymph glands can become larger and feel more tender when the body is fighting an infection.

What is lymphoedema?

Lymphoedema is a visible swelling that develops because there is a problem with the lymph drainage system. Changes in the skin and the surface tissues (*subcutaneous tissues*) can result. The lymph system is no longer able to drain away all the fluid and waste products that have built up in the tissues. The swelling that develops when the lymph system cannot work properly is not just made up of fluid but also contains material such as fat cells. In time, the skin can lose its soft feeling and become hard due to fibrous changes (*fibrosis*), or rubbery because of the build-up of fat cells. The swelling is usually in an arm or leg, although it can affect more than one part of the body. It is often described as 'chronic oedema' because the swelling has been present for many months or years. A few people have a *midline* lymphoedema (see page 45). Sometimes the face, breast or genitals can be swollen.

There may be a known reason why the lymph drainage channels become damaged or blocked. When there is a known external cause for the failure it is called a *secondary lymphoedema*. Sometimes the swelling is cancer-related, but there can be non-cancer-related causes.

Non-cancer-related causes of swelling

- accidental injury that damages the lymphatic system
- infection of the skin and tissues
- poor blood drainage through the veins
- inability to exercise or move the limb

Cancer-related causes of swelling

- cancer or cancer treatment, for example surgery to remove lymph nodes, or radiotherapy to the lymph nodes

There is a risk of lymphoedema when the cancer treatment has affected the lymph nodes in the neck, armpits or groin, for example:

- breast cancer
- gynaecological cancer
- melanoma (a type of skin cancer)
- prostate cancer
- sarcoma (a cancer of muscle, connective tissue or fat)

In most cases lymphoedema develops soon after treatment, but swelling may appear many years afterwards. The reason is not known, but sometimes it can be triggered by a skin infection (*cellulitis*). If there is no apparent reason for the swelling it is usual to carry out further tests to make sure that there is no new medical problem.

Lymphoedema can be diagnosed in people who have not had cancer treatment and where there is no obvious cause. *Primary lymphoedema* is a term used to describe swelling that usually happens because the lymph vessels have not developed properly. Some people are born without enough lymph vessels, whereas others have very large leaky vessels that do not work well. It can affect men, women and children at any age and at any time.

The genetic characteristics of some forms of inherited lymph-oedema can now be identified. Despite this new information, it is still not easy to determine why this is a problem that affects some people but not others.

Lipoedema – often confused with lymphoedema

Lipoedema is a disorder of fat. It mainly affects women and starts in adolescence or other times of hormonal change, such as pregnancy. The condition leads to swelling around the buttocks, thighs and legs and sometimes the arms. The leg swelling often finishes around the ankles, while the feet stay a normal shape. The hands and upper body are often normal. The skin is tender when pressed and bruises easily. Dieting does not usually help to reduce the swelling, even when there is weight loss from other parts of the body such as face, neck and chest.

Women who have had lipoedema for some years can also develop lymphoedema, which is called *lipoedema with lymphoedema*.

How many people have lymphoedema?

It is estimated that around 100,000 people in the UK suffer with chronic swelling. Most of the information is about people with a breast cancer related lymphoedema. It appears that one in every four women who have had breast cancer will have a lifetime risk of developing some degree of swelling, although this is usually mild (in 90% of cases). There is some evidence that new breast cancer surgery, such as sentinel node biopsy, is likely to reduce the number of people who develop lymphoedema.

A recent study suggests that chronic oedema is more of a problem in older people. Around one in 200 people over the age of 65 is affected, and in most cases (75%) the swelling is not related to cancer.

HOW TREATMENT CAN HELP

Appropriate treatment can help to reduce and control lymphoedema by improving the lymph drainage from the swollen area. Healthy lymph vessels are stimulated to work better, and new drainage pathways open up. Many of the problems caused by lymphoedema can be prevented by hygiene measures to prevent skin infections.

What is the treatment?

The 'Four Cornerstones of Treatment' to help manage your condition are:

- skin care
- compression
- exercise
- massage

Sometimes the swelling is complicated and needs a more *intensive course* of treatment. This will depend on the severity of the swelling and the part of the body that is affected. An intensive course of treatment is carried out by a lymphoedema practitioner and will include:

- massage (manual lymphatic drainage)
- bandaging (multi-layer lymphoedema bandaging)

Intensive bandaging helps to reduce the swelling before *maintenance therapy* is started. Maintenance therapy is the part of treatment that helps to keep the swelling under control. If the swelling is not complicated you can begin this straight away. Once you feel confident you will be able to self-manage your lymphoedema.

You may find it takes several weeks or even months to see an improvement, especially if you have had swelling for a number of years. Even if the swelling is slow to improve, your arm or leg should start to feel more comfortable as the tissues start to soften.

You will have a lot in common with other people with lymphoedema, but it may be difficult to find someone with exactly the same problems. Each person is individual in the way that the swelling develops and how treatment can help.

If you have any questions or concerns about the information in this booklet you should speak to your doctor or a lymphoedema practitioner, if one is available in your area. The Lymphoedema Support Network (page 48) provides useful fact sheets that can help. There are some medical problems that *must* be checked out with your doctor before following any of the advice in this booklet. These are:

- swelling that appears rapidly over a few hours or days
- a limb that has suddenly become hot, red and painful
- if you know you have swelling of the legs due to poor veins

- if you know you have swelling due to a heart problem
- swelling that appears a few weeks after a surgical operation
- if you are being tested for, or if you are receiving treatment for, a blood clot

How to recognise lymphoedema

Lymphoedema is described as a chronic swelling that has been present for at least three months and does not reduce with diuretics (water tablets) or elevation. The following are often the first signs of the condition:

- the swelling may come and go
- more noticeable swelling at the end of the day
- a mild swelling of part of the limb, such as the foot or ankle
- the swollen part aches or feels tender
- the swelling is often worse in hot weather

Usually lymphoedema develops gradually and causes no discomfort. The swelling is soft at first, and if you press the skin with your finger it will leave a small indentation where you have pushed out the fluid (*pitting*). In time, the skin and soft tissues may become harder and more solid.

Problems that are not directly related to the swelling may occur. If you suffer from any of these symptoms *in or around the swollen area* it is important that you consult your GP or hospital doctor:

- sudden and severe pain
- sharp and shooting pain
- burning or extremely tender feeling
- numbness or a feeling of pins and needles
- muscle weakness

What to do if you think you have lymphoedema

Lymphoedema is only one cause of swelling and it is important to see your doctor first so that other causes can be ruled out. You may need to go for further investigations such as an X-ray or scan. The swelling can be caused by an infection of the skin (*cellulitis*), and this can be treated with antibiotics. You may have to wait some time for an appointment with a lymphoedema practitioner, but there are still some ways in which you can help yourself while you are waiting. Daily care of your skin is very important and can be started straight away.

If you have been told that there is no other medical problem that is causing your condition, you can begin to do some of the exercises described in this book. It is always important to keep exercise within comfortable limits and to *slowly* build up your level of activity. Take care about the way that you use your swollen limb, and make a point of checking your posture regularly so that you are not putting strain on any muscles or joints. Follow a diet that will keep you healthy as well as keep your weight under control (see page 42).

Your feelings

Lymphoedema can have an effect on your personal life and make you feel angry and upset. You may feel depressed and isolated, especially if you are dealing with any other problems in your life. As you get to know more about the condition and how you can help yourself, you may find that you feel more positive. There are many people with lymphoedema who share the same feelings. It can sometimes help if you are able to talk about what is troubling you. If you have family or friends who are able to help you, try to work out how they can share your work or help you with your treatment.

If you feel that you want to talk with someone outside your family or circle of friends, your lymphoedema practitioner or GP may be able to help. They will have an understanding of the sort of problems you face and may be able to suggest some solutions. You may prefer to talk to someone who also has lymphoedema. There are a number of local support groups as well as the telephone helpline offered by the Lymphoedema Support Network.

THE FOUR CORNERSTONES OF TREATMENT (1) SKIN CARE

Regular and careful skin care helps to:

- keep the skin in good condition
- prevent the skin changes that can happen with lymphoedema
- prevent infection

Swollen skin can become dry and cracked. It may feel thicker and less elastic than normal skin. Small cracks or cuts will allow germs to enter, and this can cause cellulitis.

Cellulitis

Cellulitis is an infection caused by bacteria that affects the skin and the tissues beneath it (*subcutaneous tissues*). The immune system in the swollen part of the body is not working as well and cannot fight the infection. Sometimes this problem is called an *acute inflammatory episode* (AIE). It can cause people to feel unwell, as though you are going down with flu. You may also have the following symptoms:

- red skin or a rash
- increased heat and swelling
- pain

Severe cases of cellulitis can result in fever, shivers and vomiting and must be reported to your doctor without delay, as you may need hospital treatment. Cellulitis can carry on for a number of weeks in a 'grumbling' form that can make you feel off-colour and tired, but there are no clear signs of infection. It could be that the old infection has flared up again, or it may be a new episode. If you think that you are developing an infection you need to see your doctor. It is important that you take the full course of any antibiotics that the doctor may prescribe.

If you are unwell with cellulitis, you should not continue with your exercises or massage, and do not wear your compression garment. It is better to rest and keep the arm or leg well supported and comfortable. If you are lying in bed, rest your limb on one or two pillows until the infection has settled down and you start to feel better. Although you may not feel like eating, it is still important to drink plenty of water.

If the swelling or the way you feel does not improve, you may need more antibiotics. You may need to continue with a low dose of anti-biotics over a number of years. This is called *prophylactic antibiotics.*

Fungal infections can also cause problems for people with lymphoedema. This sort of infection arises when two skin surfaces are touching and the skin is moist and warm. This can happen under the breasts or between skin folds. 'Athlete's foot' between the toes of a swollen foot can lead to cellulitis in the whole leg. You should inspect the skin daily as you wash and dry, and use an anti-fungal powder or cream in the affected area. Another precaution with athlete's foot is to wipe between each toe with surgical spirit once a day. Fungal infection can be treated with an anti-fungal cream that can be bought over the counter, although it would be wise to check with the pharmacist first.

Caring for your skin

Cellulitis is often one of the main reasons why lymphoedema develops or gets worse. Good skin care can help prevent broken or damaged skin and reduce the risk of cellulitis. Here are some ways that you can care for your skin:

- apply unperfumed moisturising cream once and if possible twice a day
- treat any cuts or grazes as soon as you can. Clean the skin well and then use antiseptic solution. If the area starts to show signs of cellulitis, arrange to see your doctor as soon as possible
- use insect repellents to prevent bites
- if you have pets, treat them to control fleas
- use high factor sunscreen (factor 15 or higher) to protect the swollen skin in sunny weather
- avoid hot water on your skin, and also saunas
- use an electric razor if shaving
- if you get cold easily, try wearing extra clothes rather than using hot water bottles or electric blankets. Use layers of clothing such as thermal vests or body warmers to keep you warm in the winter rather than sitting too close to a fire or radiator

If you have arm swelling

- protect the skin by using rubber or PVC gloves when you have your hands in water or are carrying out household chores
- thick gloves can be used for activities like gardening to avoid hand injuries

If you have leg swelling

- wear protective clothes and footwear on your legs and feet when gardening
- do not walk around barefoot
- when swimming, wear slip-on shoes when you are walking around the pool and in the changing room

THE FOUR CORNERSTONES OF TREATMENT
(2) COMPRESSION

Compression garments

Compression garments are made of a firm elasticated material. They apply pressure to the skin and provide support to reduce the swelling. Usually they are sleeves or stockings but garments are available for other parts of the body. They improve the effect of exercise by helping the muscles 'massage' fluid out through the existing lymphatic vessels. To get the best effect you will need to exercise and move your limb while wearing one. Compression garments will not work well if they do not fit properly or are old and worn. They should:

- be firm and provide enough pressure
- cover all the swollen area
- give the strongest support at the hand or foot so that fluid is pushed away from the limb and towards the centre of the body
- feel comfortable to wear

Compression garments can cause damage in people who:

- have poor circulation
- have trouble with cold hands and feet
- suffer from poor sensation

If you have any of these problems, you should ask your doctor for advice before using compression garments.

There are many different sorts of garment and it takes skill to choose and fit the one that will help you the most. Sleeves or stockings will often be provided from an off-the-shelf range, but some people have a garment made to their individual measurements. You may need to have different sorts of garment to fit your activity. This could mean a firmer garment to wear while exercising and something more lightweight for use in the evenings.

Guidelines for garments

- all the areas that are swollen should be covered. This could mean that you wear more than one garment, such as a glove and a sleeve, or a toecap with a leg stocking
- you will find it easier to put on your sleeve/stocking first thing in the morning when there is least swelling
- aim at wearing the garment all day. The swelling is likely to increase if you keep taking the sleeve or stocking off during the day
- you do not need to wear your garment at night unless advised to do so by your therapist
- you do not need to wear your garment while taking a bath or shower. It will be easier to put your garment back on again if the water is not too hot and you have dried thoroughly
- silk linings are available that help the stocking or sleeve to slide on – ask your lymphoedema therapist
- a pair of household rubber gloves will help you grip as you put the garment on and also get an even spread of material
- apply moisture cream at night after you have removed your garment

Checklist for the day when using a compression sleeve or stocking

- is the material of the sleeve or stocking spread equally along its length so that there is even pressure?
- are there any creases or wrinkles? These will act like tight elastic bands and cause fluid to build up behind them. This can also happen if you roll the top of the sleeve or stocking over. If the sleeve or stocking seems too long, use a rubber glove to ease the extra material evenly down the limb until the length is right
- is the sleeve or stocking tight and painful? If you notice that the fingers or toes turn a dusky purple or blue colour, take the garment off straight away and seek advice from the person who supplied it to you
- does the arm or leg become uncomfortable when you are wearing your garment? This may be because you are not moving your limb enough to stimulate the circulation. Try gentle exercise, and if the discomfort still persists *after twenty minutes* take the stocking or sleeve off and seek advice from your therapist

- is the sleeve or stocking too loose? If the garment is not fitting well it will not do its job. You need to go back to the person who supplied the sleeve or stocking to be re-measured
- is the garment still working well? Two sleeves worn in turn will last for around six months. Stockings may need more frequent replacement if you lead a more active lifestyle. If only one garment is used all the time it will need to be replaced at least every three months
- do you have swollen toes? Lymphoedema stockings do not treat swollen toes. You will need special toe-gloves to wear as well as your stocking

Keep garments in good condition. Regular washing helps the elastic in the material to work at its best. Check the washing instructions for details, although hand- or machine-washing on a cool wash (30°C) is usually recommended. Do not tumble-dry or place on a radiator to dry. Fabric conditioners are not usually recommended, as they can have an effect on the elastic quality of the garment. It helps to alternate your garments through the week so that the elastic material can rest and reshape before being used again.

Using clothes to support the swelling

Clothing such as sports tops or leggings that contain lycra may help to give light support to the swollen area. If you have genital swelling, you may find that lycra leggings or shorts will provide additional support between the legs and around the lower part of the abdomen. If you have swelling over part of your trunk you can also be supplied with some special compression garments that will provide stronger support.

THE FOUR CORNERSTONES OF TREATMENT (3) EXERCISE AND MOVEMENT

Exercise

Lymph flow depends on the muscles working like a pump to encourage drainage and prevent fluid from pooling.

We all exercise our muscles in different ways by just moving around and carrying out day-to-day activities. Some people enjoy taking part in recreational exercise such as walking, playing a sport or going to the gym. You may have been given special exercises to help you gain strength of movement. All the different types of exercise can be used to help your lymphoedema, as long as you follow certain guidelines. But exercise that is harder or more demanding than usual may make the swelling worse.

How to use daily activities to reduce the swelling

- it is always important to wear your compression garment when you undertake any form of exercise, so that the muscles can work more effectively
- ease off any activity when you start to feel tired and uncomfortable
- muscle action during moving and stretching activities will help to reduce the swelling
- activities where you have to hold a limb in one position can cause the swelling to increase
- if you have arm swelling, protect the skin when you are doing activities such as cooking, washing up or cleaning
- avoid carrying objects with your swollen arm
- tasks such as ironing and vacuum cleaning can put a lot of strain on the swollen side. Try to keep up with these jobs by doing a little at a time and changing hands when possible
- hand and foot exercises are easy to do and very helpful. Try to do these kinds of exercises regularly during the day (see pages 19–21)
- breathing exercises (pages 14–15) can be done at any time. These will help to improve the deep lymphatic drainage by using the diaphragm (a large muscle) to help pump the lymph so that it can drain away

How to use recreational exercise to reduce the swelling

Everyone has a different level of fitness and ability to exercise. It is important to find the right balance of activity that suits you. If you are returning to an activity that you have not done for some time, start with a short session in which you do not overstrain yourself, and then build up gradually.

- compression garments are very important during recreational activity and you may need firmer stockings or sleeves than usual
- start a new activity for a short time and see how your limb manages – then gradually build up
- it is possible to improve and increase your activity levels, but this has to be done slowly and carefully
- if you have arm swelling, some activities such as lifting weights or press-ups are to be avoided unless you have specific coaching from a physiotherapist who specialises in lymphoedema treatment
- if you want to return to more exertive activities such as running, seek the advice of a lymphoedema therapist as you may need to take special precautions
- racquet sports can increase hand swelling if you grip the racquet for long periods. Try to exercise your hand and loosen your grip between shots
- cycling and cross country walking will be helpful if you have leg swelling
- wear suitable protective clothing for your activity and have the necessary equipment to protect yourself from possible injury
- many people find that swimming and water exercise is very helpful. You do not need to be able to swim, as just exercising in the water will help
- yoga encourages you to stretch and relax and also to breathe correctly
- give yourself plenty of time to stretch all your muscles in your warm-up and cool-down sessions
- add the breathing exercise (below) into your warm-up and cool-down routines
- finish off your exercise with a warm or cool bath or shower. Do not be tempted to use the sauna as the heat may cause the swelling to increase

Breathing exercise

The diaphragm is a large sheet of muscle that stretches across the body between your chest and abdomen. Gentle deep breathing encourages the diaphragm to work, and you will notice the lower ribs and the abdomen expand as you breathe in. If possible, breathe in through your nose and sigh out through your mouth. This causes the pressures inside the chest to change, helping the deep lymph system to work better. This will in turn help the lymph to drain out of the limbs. Breathing exercises can be done at any time and should be done at the beginning and end of your self-massage and exercise routine.

To do this type of breathing, place both hands on your abdomen so that you can feel the bottom of your ribs (Fig. 2). Let your fingers touch at the front. Without arching your back, breathe in slowly and deeply. You will feel your hands move apart as your abdomen expands. Hold for a slow count of three, and then breathe out slowly while gently pressing your abdomen down with your hands. Repeat four more times.

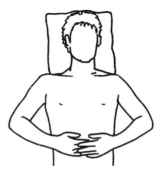

Figure 2:
Position of hands
for taking
deep breaths.

Arm exercises

These exercises are particularly useful to help keep your shoulder joints mobile and prevent stiffness. They should be done slowly so that you can concentrate on a gentle stretch. Start by doing each exercise three times and build up to five – but make sure that you do not speed up!

The exercises provided in this book can be added into your warm-up and cool-down routine if you are involved in recreational activities. They are also useful exercises to do when you are in water.

The first set of exercises, Set A, will help you to keep the shoulders mobile. The ones in Set B use the muscles in your swollen arm and stimulate lymph drainage. The exercises can be done standing, or while sitting on a stool or armless chair.

15

SET A

Shrug your shoulders up to your ears and then push them down towards the floor (Fig.3).

Figure 3:
Shoulder shrugging.

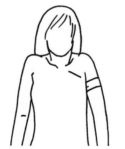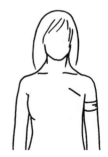

Circle your shoulders forwards and then backwards (shoulder rolls) (Fig. 4).

Figure 4:
Shoulder circling, forwards and backwards.

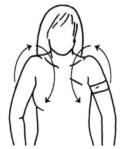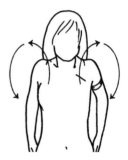

Place your hands on your shoulders. Lift your elbows out so that they are in a level line with your shoulders, hold for the count of five and then let them rest back down to your side (Fig. 5).

Figure 5:
Lifting elbows out to the side.

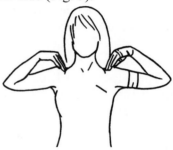

With your hands on your shoulders, bring your elbows into your sides, slowly swing the elbows forward and hold for the count of five. Now slowly swing them backwards and hold the elbows stretched back for another count of five before bringing them to rest at your side (Fig. 6).

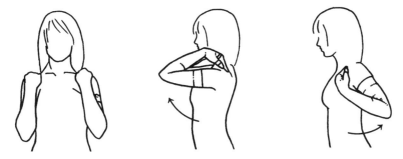

Figure 6: Hands on shoulders, elbows by side. Stretching elbows forwards and then backwards.

Place your hands behind your head and try to stretch your elbows apart as much as possible. Hold for the count of five, then slowly stretch your arms so that your hands reach down in front of the body, and then reach them behind your back (Fig 7).

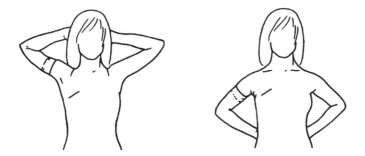

Figure 7: Hands behind head, elbows stretching out. Then hands behind back.

Clasp your hands together and lift your arms straight up as far as they will go. Do not stretch beyond the point that is comfortable. Hold for the count of five before slowly bringing your hands down (Fig.8).

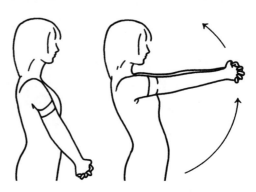

Figure 8:
Hands grasped and arms straight, ready to stretch up in the air.

When you are able to move your arms comfortably above your shoulders, try the following exercises.

Stretch your arms in front of you at shoulder level. Do the breast-stroke movement slowly and try to stretch out as far as you can (Fig. 9).

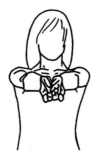

Figure 9:
Breast-stroke movement.

With the swollen arm, point to the floor just in front of your feet. Keeping your arm straight, stretch it up in the air and up over the back of your head, then back to your side. It is like painting rainbows with your fingertips. Try to stretch more each time you repeat this exercise (Fig. 10, opposite page).

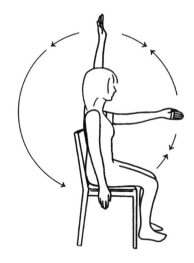

Figure 10:
Stretch straight arm in a
half circle.

SET B

Bend your arm at the elbow, then straighten it slowly. If your arm is
heavy, support it at the elbow by resting it on a flat surface (Fig. 11).

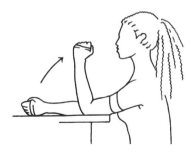

Figure 11:
Rest the elbow on a surface.
Bend and stretch the arm at
the elbow.

Bend and stretch your hand at the wrist so that your finger tips point to
the ceiling and then to the floor (Fig. 12).

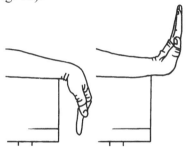

Figure 12:
Rest the forearm on a
surface. Exercise the wrist by
pointing to the ceiling and
then to the floor.

Slowly spread out your fingers and hold for the count of five, then make a fist (Fig. 13).

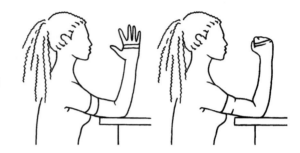

Figure 13:
Rest the elbow on a surface, make a fist, then stretch the fingers out.

Leg exercises

The sort of exercise that you can do will depend on your age and level of fitness. It is important to stay within a range that is comfortable and which does not cause you to strain.

The exercises in Set C help you to use the calf muscles to pump fluid out of the legs. They can be repeated often during the day, and each exercise should be repeated five times. You can do the exercises either lying or else sitting with your leg supported off the floor.

If you are mobile and able to walk and move around with ease, you can try the more vigorous exercises described in Set D. These will help to keep your joints mobile and also exercise the muscles that help with lymph drainage. The best position to do the exercises described in set D is to lie on the bed or floor.

SET C

Slowly move your ankle so that you bend your foot up and stretch the back of your legs. Hold for the count of five and then slowly point the toes to stretch at the ankle, and again hold for the count of five (Fig. 14).

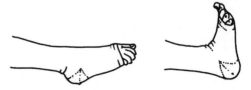

Figure 14:
Bend and stretch the foot at the ankle.

Slowly rotate your swollen foot at the ankle, making circular movements with pointed toes. First clockwise and then anti-clockwise (Fig. 15).

Figure 15:
Circle the foot in
each direction.

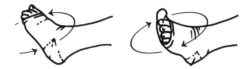

Even if you have difficulty in moving around, it is still important to move as much as you can to keep the joints supple and the muscles as strong as possible. As well as the foot exercises, you can try the following exercise when sitting in a chair or on the side of a bed (Fig. 16).

Bend your knee as far as you can and then as you stretch your leg out straight, try to work the muscles at the front of your thigh so that they feel firm. It sometimes helps to bend your ankle and pull your toes up as you work to straighten your knee. Hold the thigh muscles for the count of ten and then relax for the count of ten before starting again.

Figure 16:
Bend and stretch
the leg at the knee.

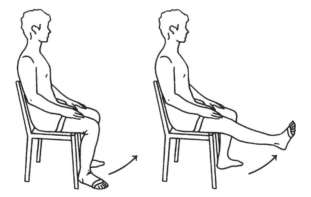

SET D

Start with your leg straight while lying on your back. Now bend your leg at the knee and then at the hip, so that your knee comes nearer to your body. Hold for the count of five before putting your foot down on the bed or floor and then stretch out your leg (Figs. 17, 18 & 19).

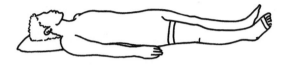

Figure 17:
Lying on your back.

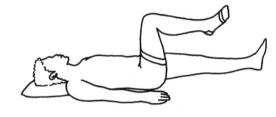

Figure 18:
Bend the swollen leg at the hip and knee.

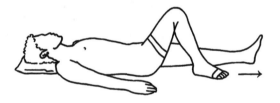

Figure 19:
Rest the foot of the bent leg on a supporting surface, then straighten at the hip and knee.

Roll over so that you are lying on the side that is not swollen. Keeping your swollen leg straight, lift it from the side so that your foot moves up towards the ceiling (Fig. 24). Hold for the count of five, then slowly lower. If both legs are swollen, then repeat on the other side.

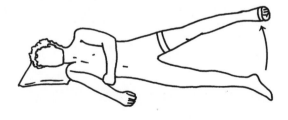

Figure 20:
Lie on the non-affected side, lift the straight swollen leg up in the air towards the ceiling.

If you are actively involved in recreational activities, make sure you combine stretching exercises in your warm-up and cool-down routine that work the muscles in your back, hips and thighs, lower legs, calves and feet. Similar activities can be done as water exercises before and after a swimming session.

Using posture and position to help

The way that you rest and move can help your lymphoedema. Good posture can help in a number of ways:

- it provides the right position for muscles to work and will help to prevent muscle strain
- it will allow you to breathe well and this in turn will help lymph drainage

Be aware of how you stand, walk and sit. Check your posture in the mirror from time to time. Make sure that your back is straight and that your shoulders are even as you sit, stand and walk. Stretch up with your head to try and make yourself taller. You should check that you are keeping your hips level by putting your hands on your hips. Make sure that you are not putting more weight on one leg than the other.

How to use position to help reduce the swelling if you have a swollen arm

- when sitting, rest your arm at shoulder height if possible and supported on a cushioned surface, otherwise rest your arm at or above heart level (Fig. 21)

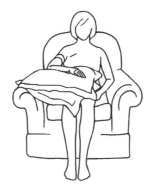

Figure 21:
Resting your swollen arm in a comfortable position so that it is at or above heart level.

- try to avoid long periods of sitting or standing without moving your arm
- make a fist, then stretch out your fingers if you are sitting and relaxing – try to do five of these every fifteen minutes
- when walking, try to wear clothes with a roomy pocket so that you are able to support your hand
- carry a small smooth pebble or squeezy ball in your pocket so that you can gently exercise your hand as you walk along
- avoid a heavy rucksack or bag straps on the swollen side, as they can restrict lymph drainage at the shoulder

How to use position to help reduce the swelling if you have a swollen leg

- rest your swollen leg at or above heart level while lying on a settee or bed, or use a recliner chair (Fig. 22)
- make sure that the full length of the leg is supported

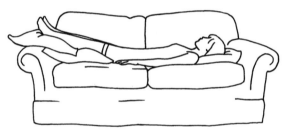

Figure 22: Resting your swollen leg in a comfortable position so that it is at or above heart level.

- some people find that sleeping with a block under the foot of the bed to raise it 5-6 centimetres will help to reduce the swelling if it is in the early stage

THE FOUR CORNERSTONES OF TREATMENT (4) MASSAGE

Manual lymphatic drainage (MLD)

This massage is used for treating lymphoedema. It is often used as part of a more intensive treatment programme and is carried out by a trained therapist. Therapists who use this technique will have a recognised qualification in one of the following methods:

- Asdonk
- Casley Smith
- Földi
- Leduc
- Vodder

MLD is not always available on the National Health Service and treatments may have to be paid for privately. A list of therapists who are skilled in these methods is available on the BLS and MLD UK websites and also through the Lymphoedema Support Network (page 48).

What does manual lymphatic drainage do?

This type of massage helps the lymph to move out of the swollen areas and into parts of the body where it can drain away normally. It stimulates new channels for the lymph to flow. This is very important when the swelling is in the body and not just in the arm or leg.

Lymphoedema massage works by clearing a pathway through the skin, so that the 'flooded' area can drain away. This usually means working on the neck and body to empty the exit routes as much as possible before starting on the arm or leg. Exercise and compression garments work by moving lymph forward ('a pushing action'). Lymphoedema massage works in a different way to other forms of treatment by drawing the lymph away ('a pulling action'). When used together, the different types of treatment will help to reduce the swelling.

There are times when you should not use massage, such as:

- during cancer treatment with radiotherapy or chemotherapy (unless directed by your doctor)
- when you have (or think you have) cellulitis
- if a limb swells suddenly

25

- if you have just been diagnosed with a blood clot in your veins (deep vein thrombosis)
- if the massage causes pain
- if you notice a sudden change in the texture or feel of the skin

In any of these cases, you need to be seen by a doctor first for further tests or treatments.

Simple lymphatic drainage (SLD – 'self massage')

Even if you have MLD from a therapist, you will need to be able to do your own massage to keep the new drainage channels working. Simple lymphatic drainage (or SLD) follows the same sequence and uses similar methods, but can be done by yourself or a carer.

The following explanation provides an introduction. You need to be shown how to do this SLD at a lymphoedema clinic or by the therapist who provides your MLD.

SLD is performed with the fingers or the flat of the hand on the skin. Your fingers are used to stretch the skin in a direction that will stimulate the lymph to flow away from the swollen part. After the skin stretch, you release the tension under your fingers so that the skin moves back. This is a very gentle movement that does not cause the skin to go red. The area should be free of oils or creams that could cause your fingers to slide too quickly. If the skin becomes sore or red during the massage it means that you are using too much pressure.

You should be in a comfortable resting position – ideally on a bed or else on a relaxing chair with your feet raised and supported. You need to be able to work easily on the lymph nodes under your arms or in the groin and not be restricted by clothing. It is important to follow the massage step by step in the order that it is described.

You should wear your compression sleeve or stocking while you do SLD to improve the effect. Deep breathing exercises are added at the beginning and end of the massage (pages 14 & 15 and Figure 23). These help to stimulate deep lymph drainage and help you relax. A family member or carer can also be shown how to do the massage. This can be very helpful if you need massage on your back.

The following description of SLD is provided to help you once you have been seen by a lymphoedema therapist. There are also self-help videos that show one way that this can be done. Further information on these videos is available from the Lymphoedema Support Network.

Simple lymphatic drainage for one arm swelling

Take five deep breaths (Fig. 23).

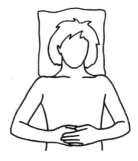

Figure 23:
Position of hands
for taking deep
breaths.

Rest your hands on each side of the neck, just below your earlobes. Stretch the skin down towards your shoulders and then release the stretch so that the skin moves back (Fig. 24). Repeat the stretch and release of skin under your fingers ten times.

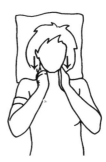

Figure 24:
Stretching the skin
at the neck.

Let your hands rest on your shoulders above your collar bones. You can do this easily if you cross your arms (Fig. 25). With flat fingers, press gently down towards the collar bone. Repeat five times.

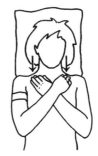

Figure 25:
Gentle pressure
above the collar
bone.

You are now ready to start work on the chest wall. To do this, you clear the lymph nodes under the armpit on the side that is not swollen. This will provide the exit route for the fluid you will move when working on the swollen side.

With the non-swollen elbow lifted slightly away from the side, apply gentle upward pressures into this armpit (Fig. 26). Do this by counting slowly to three for each pressure and then resting for the count of three before repeating. These pressures are repeated ten times.

right side swollen   *left side swollen*

Figure 26:
Gentle pressure up
into the armpit of the
non-swollen side.

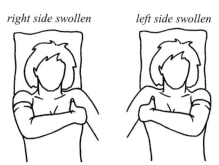

Now you can work across your body. The first hand position is on the chest on the non-swollen side near to the armpit that you have just cleared (Fig. 27). Stretch the skin towards the unaffected armpit and then release the stretch. Repeat this skin stretch ten times.

Figure 27:
Clearing the non-swollen
side.

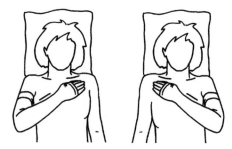

At the chest bone (sternum) in the middle of your body, continue with ten skin stretches directed towards the non-swollen armpit (Fig. 28).

Massage

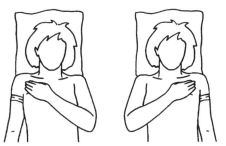

right side swollen   *left side swollen*

Figure 28:
Clearing across the
middle of the body.

You are now ready to move your hand onto the skin on the swollen side of your chest. You may need to swap hands in order to do this (Fig. 29). With your other hand, stretch the skin on the swollen side to move it in the direction of the non-swollen armpit. Repeat this ten times.

Figure 29:
Clearance of the
swollen side.

Cup your hand over the swollen shoulder and stretch the skin away from the armpit and over the top of the shoulder towards the back (Fig. 30). Repeat this ten times.

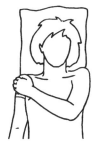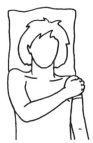

Figure 30:
Clearance over the
swollen shoulder.

Finish with five deep breaths (pages 14–15).

Simple lymphatic drainage for when you have, or when there is a risk of, swelling in both arms

There is a risk of swelling in both arms if you have had cancer in both breasts. This different method of SLD directs all drainage down to the lymph nodes in the groin. It will also be helpful if you have swelling in the upper part of your body.

Start with five deep breaths, and then clear the drainage pathways in the neck and above the collar bones on both sides, as described on page 27. You then need to work on each side of your body in turn.

Apply gentle pressure to the nodes in the groin on the right side to provide an exit route for the lymph that you will move down from the upper part of the body on this side. You can sometimes feel the groin nodes with your fingers just under the skin (Fig. 31). (The diagram on page vi shows where they are found.) Use your hand to give gentle pressures down into the groin. Do this ten times, counting slowly to three for each pressure, and then rest for the count of three before repeating.

Figure 31:
Clearance into the
groin nodes.

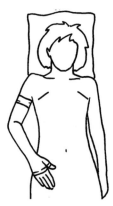

You are now ready to work over the abdomen on the right side. Start at the lower part of the abdomen and gently stretch the skin down towards your groin before letting your hands relax. Repeat this ten times. Now move your hand on to your abdomen (tummy) below your navel on the swollen side (Fig. 32). In this position, stretch the skin towards the groin and then relax your hand. Repeat ten times.

Figure 32:
Clearance at the
abdomen below the
waistline.

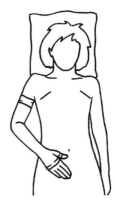

Move your hand above the navel on to the waistline (Fig. 33) and repeat ten skin stretches down towards the groin on the right side, relaxing your hands between each stretch.

Figure 33:
Clearance at the
waistline.

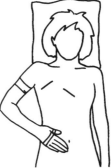

You are now ready to work above the waistline on the right chest area (Fig. 34). Repeat the ten gentle skin stretches so that you can clear the swelling down towards the groin. It is not easy to push swelling through scar lines, so make your way around them, always directing the gentle pushes towards the lymph nodes in the groin. When you have done this, apply ten gentle pressures to empty the groin lymph nodes.

Figure 34:
Clearance on the
chest.

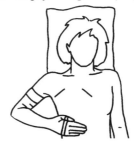

Finish off with the same SLD to the neck and above the collar bone as you started with. Do five deep breaths (page 15).

You are now ready to do the SLD again, but this time on the left side of your body.

It would help if you have a partner, friend or carer who can repeat the SLD on your back. You can clear the lymph nodes in the groin on the right side and stretch the skin towards the groin from your waist (Fig. 35). This person can then work on the right side of your back, around the waistline, and then on the chest to stretch the skin towards the groin at the front. Do this ten times in each position. Use gentle skin stretches to clear down from around the back of the chest wall. You must give feedback if you feel that the pressures are too hard or uncomfortable, as this will not help the lymph drainage. Repeat the skin stretches as described on the left side of the back.

right side swollen   *left side swollen*

Figure 35: Person helping clearance at the waist from the back.

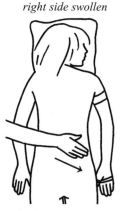
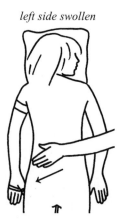

Simple lymphatic drainage for one leg swelling

Take five deep breaths (page 15).

Rest your hands on each side of the neck, just below your earlobes (Fig. 36). Stretch the skin down towards your shoulders and then release the stretch so that the skin moves back. Repeat the stretch and release of skin under your fingers ten times.

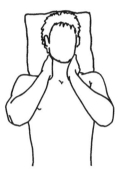

Figure 36:
Stretching the skin
at the neck.

Let your hands rest on your shoulders above your collar bones. You can do this movement easily if you cross your arms. With flat fingers, press gently down towards the collarbone (Fig. 37). Repeat this five times.

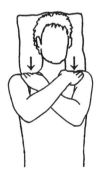

Figure 37:
Gentle pressure
above the collar
bones.
Note: No sleeves
on arms.

Now repeat the whole of this sequence two more times.

You are now ready to start work on your body. Apply gentle upward pressures into the armpit on the swollen side. This will provide the exit route for the fluid from the swollen leg. With the elbow lifted a little way from the side, massage gently upwards into the armpit (Fig. 38). Do this ten times, counting slowly to three for each pressure, and then rest for the count of three before repeating.

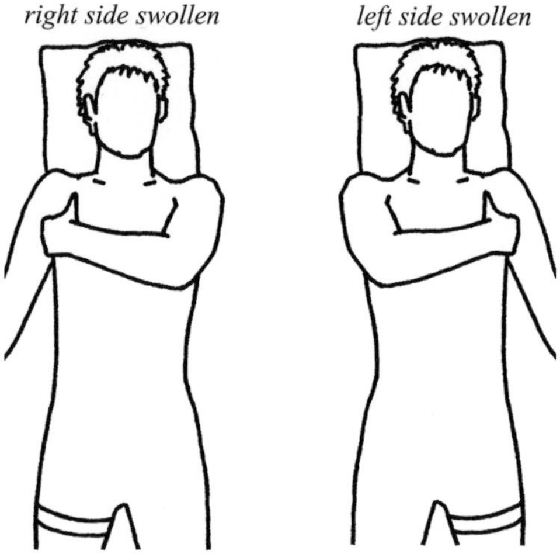

right side swollen   *left side swollen*

Figure 38:
Gentle pressure into
armpit on the
swollen side.

Lower your hand to rest it below the armpit on the chest wall on the swollen side, just above your waist (Fig. 39). Stretch the skin up towards the armpit you have just cleared. Repeat this skin stretch ten times and relax between each stretch.

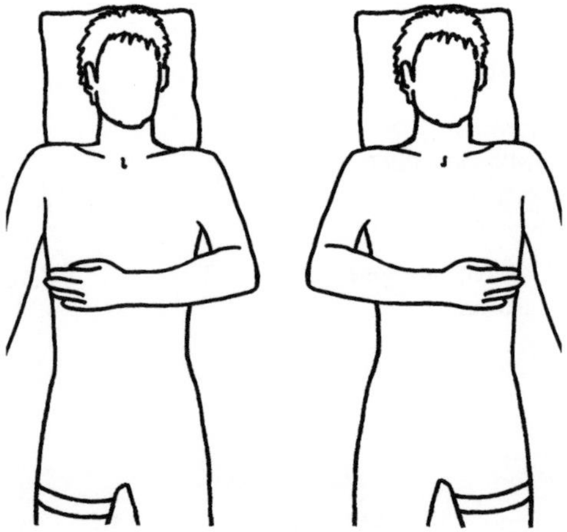

Figure 39:
Clearance of chest
on the swollen side.

When you reach the waistline, repeat the upward skin stretches ten times to help the drainage up to the armpit (Fig. 40).

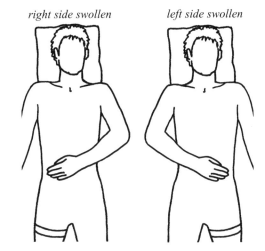

right side swollen   *left side swollen*

Figure 40:
Clearance over waist
on the swollen side.

You can now work over the abdomen and hip on the side of the swelling (Fig. 41). Use upward skin stretches to direct the flow from the abdomen towards the armpit on the same side. Do this ten times over the abdomen and then ten times up the side of the body, from the hip towards the armpit.

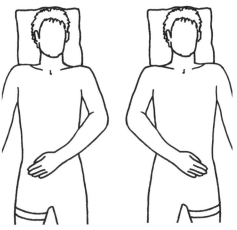

Figure 41:
Clearance over
abdomen on the
swollen side.

Finish with five deep breaths (page 15).

As shown on page 32, it will help if you have a partner, friend or carer who can repeat the SLD on your back. You can clear the lymph nodes in the armpit on the swollen side (page 29) and stretch the skin towards the armpit from your waist. The other person can then help with clearance at the waist and below on the swollen side from the back, and stretch the skin up towards the armpit (Fig. 42). This is repeated ten times in each position. Use gentle skin stretches to clear up to the armpit on the swollen side from around the waist and buttocks. You must give feedback if you feel that the pressures are too hard or uncomfortable, as this will not help the lymph drainage.

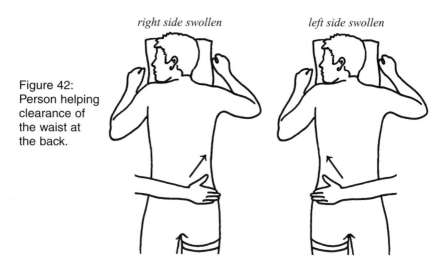

right side swollen   *left side swollen*

Figure 42:
Person helping
clearance of
the waist at
the back.

Simple lymphatic drainage for when you have, or when there is a risk of, swelling in both legs

When you have swelling in both legs you need to work on each side of the body in turn, using the drainage pathways up to the armpit for one side and then the other. This SLD method will also be helpful if you have swelling in the lower part of the trunk or in the genital area. Start the SLD on each side in turn by working on both sides of the neck and above the collar bone (page 33). Do five deep breathing exercises before you begin and at the end of the SLD for each leg.

Skin brushing

You can use a skin brush instead of your hands to do some or all of the massage. Skin brushes are available from a number of retail outlets. Choose a brush that is comfortable to use and which causes the skin to wrinkle as you brush, without causing it to become red or sore. It is worth trying different types of brush to find one that you like and which works well for you.

Sometimes you may be advised by your lymphoedema therapist to use an electrical body massager. If this is the case, use the weakest setting with a dimpled head and always use the heat-free option. Anything that heats the skin may increase the swelling. Let the massager rest on the skin without pressing and work around each area in small circles. Read the manufacturer's instructions carefully before using. You can use the sequence described in this section for your type of swelling.

INTENSIVE TREATMENT

When intensive treatment is needed it will usually mean daily treatment provided by a trained lymphoedema therapist. It usually takes between two to three weeks to complete this treatment. At the end of intensive treatment you will be fitted with a compression garment, and maintenance therapy can start. Intensive treatment is sometimes called by other names:

- decongestive lymphatic therapy (DLT)
- combined physical therapy (CPT)
- complex decongestive therapy (CDT)

All these names describe the same treatment, which consists of:

- care of the skin
- manual lymphatic drainage (MLD)
- bandaging of the limb (multi-layer lymphoedema bandaging – MLLB)
- exercise programme

Some clinics also use compression pumps as part of intensive treatment (see page 39).

If the swelling is slight and causes no problems you will probably not need intensive treatment. Mild lymphoedema can be well controlled using the four types of self-treatment that have already been described.

Intensive treatment is needed if there are complications such as:
- a large swelling
- a limb that has swollen out of shape
- skin that is not in good condition
- a solid swelling

Before you start, your therapist will give you information about what to expect and also what you need to bring with you. Although many people find this treatment very helpful they can also find it very tiring, so be prepared to take things easy during the treatment period. It is also likely that you will need to make arrangements for travelling to your appointments, as driving can be very difficult in your bandages. If you do intend to drive yourself, it is a good idea to check first with your car insurance company to be certain that this will not invalidate your insurance cover.

As intensive treatment is a lengthy and time-consuming process you may have to wait some time before you can be treated. There are some parts of the UK where this type of treatment is not readily available. The British Lymphology Society (BLS) and the LSN provide information about treatment centres and their contact details (page 48).

Multi-layer lymphoedema bandaging (MLLB)

MLLB works to reduce the swelling and improve the shape of the limb by helping the muscles pump fluid out. The bandage is made up of a number of layers including:
- a tube of light cotton (stockinette) next to the skin
- padding which can be made of cotton or foam
- hard foam, which is sometimes used to shape the limb
- layers of non-elastic bandages

The bandages should feel comfortable and not constrictive. They help the muscles to pump the fluid out of the limb by causing changes in pressures. High pressures build up during exercise, compared with low pressures at rest.

The bandages are applied every day and remain in place overnight. Usually bandages are not changed over the weekend, although you may be shown how to bandage yourself so that you can replace any loose or uncomfortable bandages. Bandages that are uncomfortable or causing a constriction should be taken off. If you are able to self-bandage you can reapply, or else you can put on your compression garment until you go back to the clinic.

Bandages can help to treat swelling in other parts of the body. An example of this is swelling in the penis and scrotum, where small and softer bandages are used. You will be shown how to do this sort of bandaging so that you can change it frequently.

Specially-designed support body garments can also be used to help swollen parts of the body. These can be supplied by your lymph-oedema clinic or the surgical appliance department at your hospital.

OTHER TREATMENTS

Compression pumps

This a small pump attached by plastic tubing to an inflatable tube that fits on your arm or leg. The pump is powered from the mains and pumps air into an inflatable tube. When the machine is switched on, the tube will inflate and then go down for a few minutes before inflating again.

There are times when limb swelling can be helped by using a compression pump. This does not replace the other sorts of treatment and you still need to wear your sleeve or stocking. You should always check with your doctor or a lymphoedema specialist before you decide to buy or use a compression pump. If you are advised to use one, the treatment pressure setting should never be greater than 40 mmHg. Pressures over this level could damage the fragile lymph vessels near the surface of the skin.

There are times when a compression pump should not be used, and these are:

- if you have heart problems
- if you have swelling that has suddenly appeared and you have not seen a doctor about this

- when the swelling is on the body as well as in the arm or leg
- if there is swelling in the breast or genital area
- if you have cellulitis
- if using the pump is painful. In these cases the use of a pump may make the lymphoedema worse, so always seek advice before use

The use of drugs to treat lymphoedema

Antibiotics are often recommended within your treatment programme to treat cellulitis. Apart from this sort of treatment, tablets are not usually used to treat lymphoedema.

Sometimes people are prescribed diuretics (water tablets) that work by causing the body to dehydrate. Although they can help with some types of swelling, they do not help to improve lymph drainage. Powerful diuretics can cause harm if taken for a long period without medical supervision.

Benzopyrones (e.g. Coumarin) have also been used to treat lymphoedema. However, there is little evidence to show that these drugs are effective for the condition.

The use of surgery for lymphoedema

Different types of surgery have been used around the world. People who have had surgery will still need to continue with the four corner-stones of treatment, including the use of a compression garment. The different sorts of surgical treatment include:

Reducing or debulking surgery

This involves removing the swollen skin and tissues from the limb. This surgery is useful for swelling in certain parts of the body such as the scrotum, penis or eyelids. It is only an option for arm or leg swelling when all other treatments have failed. This treatment involves major operations that should only be performed by specialist surgeons.

Microsurgery

Microsurgery produces a new drainage channel for the lymph by making new connections between parts of the lymph system or the veins. There are only a few centres around the world that provide it. At the time of writing, lymphatic micorsurgery is not available in the UK.

Liposuction

A centre in Sweden has developed a liposuction technique to treat lymphoedema. There is improvement in the swelling as long as the person continues to wear their sleeve or stocking day and night.

LIVING WITH LYMPHOEDEMA

Some questions you may ask:

My swollen limb feels heavy and uncomfortable. Is this usual?

Swelling can often cause a feeling of tightness, heaviness or a deep ache in the muscles. If the swelling is recent, it may feel tender or bruised.

- if you develop any of the symptoms described under 'Acute Inflammatory Episode' on page 8 it is important that you see your GP or hospital doctor

What should I wear?

Loose-fitting clothes with broad straps will help lymph drainage and enable you to move freely. Cotton or natural fibres are comfortable to wear and allow the air to circulate around your skin. Avoid anything that will rub and damage the skin. Certain styles of clothes will help to make the swelling less obvious. The cut and design of the clothes can be used to disguise the swollen limb.

When you have lymphoedema the body will need to use drainage pathways that are near to the skin surface. Avoid wearing:

- underwear with tight elastic or narrow bands
- elasticated cuffs to sleeves and socks
- tight jewellery, including rings and watches
- bras with narrow straps or underwire supports

If you have a swollen leg, footwear is very important. The following suggestions may help:

- a shoe with a low heel and which supports the foot will help you to walk with more comfort and confidence

- a lace-up shoe or boot provides support to the foot and helps to reduce the swelling, as it acts to massage the tissues during movement
- court shoes or sandals allow fluid to bulge on top of the foot and between the straps. Although they may feel easy to put on, they can cause the swelling to increase in the foot
- poorly-fitting shoes can cause blistering and rubbing of the skin
- walking barefoot should be avoided, as it increases the risk of damaging the skin and also of picking up infection
- wear slip-on shoes to protect your feet when walking around swimming pools and changing areas
- certain footwear can make the foot become hot and sticky. This increases the risk of fungal infections, such as athlete's foot
- try to find a pair of indoor and outdoor shoes that are comfortable so that you can change your footwear during the day

(The Lymphoedema Support Network also has a useful factsheet on swollen feet.)

Is diet important?

Swelling is more difficult to control if you are overweight, because the fluid cannot move easily through fat tissue. As a general rule, your waist circumference should be less than, or the same as, half your height. You can also check your body weight, although this will increase if you have a lot of swelling. The best way to keep your weight under control is to follow a normal healthy diet:

- reduce the amount of processed foods
- eat plenty of fresh fruit and vegetables
- water and fruit juices are a better alternative to tea, coffee and sugary drinks

In addition, people with lymphoedema should be aware of the following:

- restricting your water intake is not recommended. This will not help to reduce the lymphoedema, and could be harmful
- although there is no evidence to suggest that lymphoedema is related to salt in the diet, a reduction of salt has been recommended as a general health guidance

- certain foods and drinks (such as alcohol and spicy foods) can increase swelling in some people

You can also get useful healthy-eating factsheets from your GP surgery or the LSN.

What can I do in hot weather?

When you are warm the skin may become pink and puffy, because more blood flows to the skin surface to help you cool down. This is likely to cause more swelling. To prevent more swelling in hot weather, you can:

- wear your sleeve or stocking, as this will resist the increase in fluid. Although you may not feel like wearing your garment when it is hot, this is the time when you most need to!
- ask about choices of compression garment, as some are made with an open weave which may be cooler to wear
- avoid vigorous exercise during the hot part of the day
- avoid going out in the midday heat and try to stay in the shade
- when relaxing, try to rest your swollen limb at or just above heart level

Should I make any special arrangements to travel?

Long journeys may increase the swelling because you are not able to move and stimulate lymph drainage. There are ways that you can help yourself:

- get up for short walks if on a train or aeroplane
- take frequent stops if you are travelling in a motor vehicle
- simple exercises that you can do at any time include moving your shoulders, squeezing and stretching your fingers, or bending and stretching your foot
- drink plenty of water. The amount of water drunk does not increase lymphoedema swelling

If on an aeroplane flight

- wear your compression sleeve or stocking and do any of the exercises that can be undertaken in the space that is available to you
- try to arrange to have a seat where you have more space and may be able to get your swollen limb raised

- rest your arm on a couple of flight pillows to one side rather than keeping your arm across the body
- ask your GP or your lymphoedema therapist to write a letter to the flight company to support your request for a suitable seat.

Does it matter what position I sleep in?

- it is important that you go to bed in order to sleep and rest. Sleeping in a chair can cause fluid to pool in the limbs, and this will increase the swelling
- avoid a sleeping position with your swollen arm tucked underneath your body, as this may restrict lymph drainage
- sometimes your therapist will suggest that you bandage your limb overnight. In this case, make sure you are clear about how to apply the bandages and that you have all the equipment you need

SPECIAL NEEDS

Lymphoedema in children and teenagers

Having a baby or young child with lymphoedema can be an anxious and frustrating time. There is often little information and parents struggle to find a diagnosis and treatment. Fortunately lymphoedema in children is rare, but this means that there are only a small number of professionals with the experience to help. The lymphoedema can have certain features:

- the swelling can be in more than one part of the body
- birthmarks such as a port-wine stain may also be present
- there may be other unusual features affecting the shape and dimensions of parts of the body

The usual cause is a failure of the proper development of the lymph drainage route, with either too few lymph vessels or a system that has not properly developed. Sometimes lymph vessels develop late, in which case swelling can disappear as the child grows.

Although lymphoedema does not usually create too many problems for the child, the consequences of the condition become more traumatic in teenage years. Treatment of lymphoedema in children and young people is difficult and requires special expertise. The same principles of skin care, exercise and massage apply, but compression garments will need to be made to measure and replaced regularly as the child grows.

In addition to the physical aspects of treatment, parents and young people will need access to other support and healthcare services to help them to come to terms with the condition and its effects.

Midline lymphoedema

Midline lymphoedema describes swelling in one or more of the following areas:

- head and neck
- chest
- breasts
- abdomen
- lower back
- hips
- genitals

Midline swelling is not as common as lymphoedema in the arms or legs. It is sometimes a problem in people who have primary lymphoedema. Swelling which appears in the body after an operation will often resolve after some weeks, although a few people may need special help. It is not as easy to use exercises and compression garments because of the position of the swelling. MLD is often the most useful treatment, and you will be shown how to do SLD so that you are also able to help self-manage your condition.

Swelling in your body, and especially around the genital area, may affect how you feel about yourself and your relationship with your partner. Professional advice from your GP, consultant and lymphoedema therapist may help you to address the physical or sexual problems relating to your swelling.

Breast lymphoedema

The breast can swell following treatment for breast cancer, causing it to feel heavy and uncomfortable. A firm and supportive bra that is seamless will improve comfort and support the swollen tissues. Without good support the increased weight pulls the breast down, leading to further pooling of fluid. Broad straps are important so that the weight of the breast can be spread over a wide area and avoid constriction.

Swelling in the shoulder or groin

This problem can be present if you have arm or leg lymphoedema, and means that there is a blockage at the root of the limb. If untreated it will restrict the drainage out of the arm or leg. MLD and SLD are helpful treatments, and care should be taken so that a compression garment will not cause any more swelling in this area.

Lymphoedema of the face

Facial swelling can develop after:

- injury
- infection
- certain skin disorders such as acne and rosacea

It is likely that your GP will first wish to control any inflammation with medication before any attempt is made to treat the lymphoedema. There are some ways that may help to reduce the swelling:

- anything that causes you to flush will increase the blood flow to the face and increase the swelling. For this reason, you may need to avoid alcohol, hot drinks, spicy food and hot rooms
- facial swelling can be worse after a night's sleep, because lying in a horizontal position makes the fluid pool more in the face. This can be a particular problem around the eyelids. You can help yourself by keeping your bedroom cool at night and by raising the head of the bed by 8-10 centimetres. This can be done by using blocks under the head end of the bed or by placing a pillow under the mattress
- if your face is swollen when you wake up, try standing in front of a mirror and exercise your facial muscles by making different expressions
- MLD and SLD are useful ways to treat this problem

Lymphoedema of the genitals

Genital swelling can sometimes be a problem, but is rare. Regular skin care routines are very important for people who have lymphoedema in this part of the body, as there is a risk of infection. The best way to treat this problem is MLD and SLD and to wear supportive underwear. There are some special supports and garments that can help, and your lymphoedema therapist will be able to advise you about this. The LSN has a useful fact sheet on genital lymphoedema.

CONCLUSION: TAKING CONTROL

The most important part of treatment is to give you information about what can be done to control your lymphoedema. You should feel confident that you have enough information to give you:

- a proper diagnosis
- an explanation of why you have this problem
- knowledge about the lymph system
- an understanding of how the different parts of treatment will help you
- what will help and what will make things worse

In time you will gain confidence and be efficient in your self-treatment. Your lymphoedema practitioner will stay involved if you need new sets of compression garments and will be an important contact if you need further advice and help.

Lymphoedema treatment is about how to help you to take control of the swelling. The aim is for you to become the expert in your own treatment. By making the advice given in this book a part of your daily activity you will be able to control the swelling and its effects.

USEFUL SOURCES OF INFORMATION

UK
Breast Cancer Care, Kiln House, 210 New Kings Road, London SW6 4NZ. Tel: 0207384 2984. www.breastcancercare.org.uk

British Lymphology Society, P.O. Box 196, Shoreham, Sevenoaks, Kent TN13 9BF. Tel: 01959 525524. www.lymphoedema.org/bls

Cancerbackup, 3 Bath Place, Rivington Street, London EC2A 3JR. Tel: 020 7696 9003. www.cancerbackup.org.uk

Cancer Research UK, P.O. Box 123, Lincoln's Inn Fields, London WC2A 3PX. Tel: 020 7242 0200. www.imperialcancer.co.uk

Disabled Living Foundation, 380-384 Harrow Road, London W9 2HU. Tel: 020 7289 6111. www.dlf.org.uk

Lymphoedema Support Network, St Luke's Crypt, Sydney Street, London SW3 6NH. Tel: 020 7351 0990. Fax: 020 7349 9809. adminlsn@lymphoedema.freeserve.co.uk. www.lymphoedema. org/lsn

Macmillan Cancer Relief, 89 Albert Embankment, London SE1 7UQ. Tel (freephone): 0808 808 2020. www.macmillan.org.uk

Marie Curie Cancer Care, 89 Albert Embankment, London SE1 7TP. Tel: 020 7599 7777. www.mariecurie.org.uk

MLD UK (Manual Lymphatic Drainage), P.O. Box 14491, Glenrothes KY6 3YE. Tel: 01592 840799. info@mlduk.org.uk. www.mlduk.org.uk

Australia
Lymphoedema Association of Victoria, P.O. Box 83, Ashburton, Vic., Australia. Tel: 1300 852 850. info@lavorg.au. www.lav.org.au

Canada
Lymphovenous Canada, 8 Silver Ave, Toronto, Ont. M6R 1X8, Canada. www.lymphovenous-canada.ca

Ireland
Lymphoedema Ireland, c/o The Irish Cancer Society, 43/45 Northumberland Road, Dublin 4, Ireland. Tel (freephone): 1800 200 700 info@lymphireland.com. www.lymphireland.com

New Zealand
LSN (Auckland), 15 Hillsborough Road, Mount Roskill, Auckland, New Zealand. Tel: 09 625 6463. lymphoedema.info@nzord.org.nz. www.nzord.org.nz

USA
National Lymphedema Network Inc., Latham Square, 1611 Telegraph Avenue, Suite 1111 Oakland, CA 94612-2138, USA. Tel: 510-208-3200. www.lymphnet.org

UK SUPPLIERS

Activa Healthcare Ltd, 1 Lancaster Park, Newborough Road, Needwood, Burton-on-Trent DE13 9PD. Tel: 01283 540957. Fax: 01283 576808. advice@activahealthcare.co.uk. www.activahealthcare.co.uk
Bauerfeind UK, Phyllis House, 229 Bristol Road, Birmingham B5 7UB. Tel: 0121 446 5353. Fax: 0121 446 5454. info@bauerfeind.co.uk
BSN Medical Ltd, P.O. Box 258, Willerby, Hull HU10 6WT. Tel: 01482 673583. Fax: 01482 670111. www.bsnmedical.com
Centromed Ltd, Anglo House, Wotton Road, Kingsnorth Industrial Estate, Ashford TN23 6LN. Tel: 01233 635353. Fax: 01233 635351. sales@centromed.com. www.centromed.com
Cosyfeet, The Tanyard, Leigh Road, Street BA16 0HR. Tel: 01458 447275. Fax: 01485 445988. comfort@cosyfeet.co.uk. www.cosyfeet.com
Credenhill Ltd, 10 Cossal Industrial Estate, Ilkeston DE7 5UG. Tel: 0115 932 0144. Fax: 0115 944 0437. sales@credenhill.co.uk. www.credenhill.co.uk
Haddenham Healthcare, Crendon House, Crendon Industrial Park, Long Crendon HP18 9BB. Tel: 01844 208842. Fax: 01844 208843. sales@hadhealth.com. www.hadhealth.com
Juzo UK Ltd, Unit 1, Edison Place, Dryburgh Industrial Estate, Dundee DD2 3QU. Tel: 01382 826620. Fax: 01382 826641. sales@juzo.co.uk. www.juzo.com
Medi UK Ltd, Plough Lane, Hereford HR4 0EL. Tel: 01432 373500. Fax: 01432 373510. enquiries@mediuk.co.uk. www.mediuk.co.uk
Sigvaris Britain Ltd, Unit 6A, The Foundry, London Road, Winchester SO23 7QN. Tel: 01962 886226. Fax: 01962 886212. www.sigvaris.com
Vernon Carus Ltd, 1 Western Avenue, Matrix Park, Buckshaw Village, Chorley PR7 7NB. Tel: 01772 299900. Fax: 01772 299901. mail@vernon-carus.co.uk. www.vernon-carus.co.uk

IMPORTANT LOCAL NAMES AND CONTACT DETAILS

_____

_____

_____

_____

_____

_____

_____

_____

_____

_____

_____

_____

_____

_____

_____

_____

_____

_____

_____

_____

_____

_____